E2LXG

Hysterectomy and HRT

Gautam Khastgir MD FRCS MRCOG
*Senior Registrar in
Reproductive Medicine*

John Studd DSc MD FRCOG
Consultant Gynaecologist

*Chelsea and Westminster Hospital
London, UK*

MARTIN DUNITZ

© Martin Dunitz Ltd 1998

First published in the United Kingdom
in 1998 by
Martin Dunitz Ltd
The Livery House
7– 9 Pratt Street
London NW1 0AE

A CIP record for this book is available
from the British Library.

ISBN 1-85317-408-4

Printed and bound in Spain by Cayfosa

Contents

Introduction

Hysterectomy is one of the most common gynaecological operations, with over 60 000 cases being performed in the United Kingdom every year.[1] It is an effective treatment that can permanently cure heavy painful periods, chronic pelvic pain and pre-menstrual syndrome,[2] bringing great relief to patients suffering from these debilitating conditions and improving their quality of life.[3,4] As hysterectomy is usually performed for symptom relief rather than as a life-saving procedure, it is important to ensure that patients' well-being is not jeopardized by any complication of surgery. Ovarian hormone deficiency is one such consequence of hysterectomy that may affect the quality of life. Hormone replacement therapy (HRT) should therefore be considered following hysterectomy to prevent several short- and long-term health problems.

Ovarian function

As the majority of hysterectomies are performed in the age range of 40–49 years, declining ovarian function may precede surgery. Oestrogen and testosterone deficiencies are inevitable if bilateral oophorectomy is performed, but may also occur as a result of the premature failure of conserved ovaries.[5,6] The increased possibility of ovarian failure is supported by the higher incidence and increased severity of vasomotor symptoms in hysterectomized women, who are also more likely to develop other less typical features of ovarian failure such as psychological symptoms and sexual problems. There is also a high incidence of cardiovascular disease and osteoporosis as a result of long-term oestrogen deficiency following bilateral oophorectomy, and the incidence is moderately increased even after hysterectomy with ovarian conservation.

Apart from women undergoing bilateral oophorectomy, it is impossible to predict who are at a higher risk of ovarian failure following hysterectomy. It is therefore important to monitor ovarian function in the postoperative period. HRT should be started immediately after surgery, if the ovaries are removed, or following confirmation of compromised residual ovarian function. This would improve patients' satisfaction with hysterectomy by relieving the climacteric symptoms that are often considered as complications of the surgical treatment. Hysterectomized women are ideal candidates for HRT, owing to the absence of cyclical withdrawal bleeding and progestogenic side-effects,[7] and so this group is best placed to receive its long-term health benefits.

The need for HRT

In spite of the well-recognized need for HRT, at present few hysterectomized women actually receive the treatment. Climacteric complaints are usually ignored in young women with residual ovaries and, in the absence of menstruation, diagnosis of ovarian failure is often missed. There is rarely any protocol for regular follow-up to check hormone levels in these women despite the higher risk of premature menopause. More worryingly HRT is often not advised even after bilateral oophorectomy, and when HRT is started it is taken for only a short period of time due to lack of follow-up.[8] The low uptake and continuation rates are also partly due to widespread misconceptions among both women and their doctors about the risks associated with HRT.[9]

Ovaries are removed in 20% of hysterectomies, and in a quarter of the remaining cases the conserved ovaries fail prematurely. HRT is therefore necessary in at least 40% of all hysterectomized women (Figure 1). One in five women in the UK is likely to have a hysterectomy before the age of 60.[1] The prospect of ovarian hormone deficiency in nearly half of these women indicates the size of the problem. The task of identifying and arranging HRT for such a large population seems phenomenal, but in a general practice serving a population of 2000 there would only be 50–60 hysterectomized women. These women may be easily identified as they are the women excluded from the cervical smear recall list. A protocol of annual plasma follicle stimulating hormone (FSH) and oestradiol estimations in these women would identify the need for HRT and have a great impact on their future health.

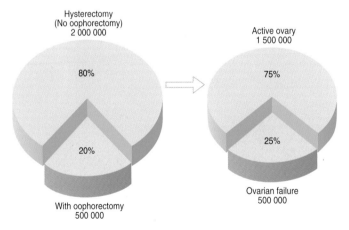

Figure 1
Number and proportion of hysterectomized women requiring HRT in the UK.

In the following chapters we discuss the different aspects of HRT following hysterectomy:

- The endocrinological changes following hysterectomy with or without oophorectomy emphasize the specific need for HRT in these women

- Unopposed oestrogen replacement is adequate for the majority but there is a strong case for testosterone replacement after bilateral oophorectomy

- It is important to appreciate that the dose of HRT has to be individualized as the dose needed may be higher in a younger woman than after natural menopause

- The short-term benefits such as relief from climacteric symptoms, improved mental health and unchanged or improved sexuality, all result in a higher rate of patient satisfaction.

- An appropriate selection of the type of HRT and routine follow-up may help to improve the long-term compliance that is needed for preventing cardiovascular disease and osteoporosis

- Risk-benefit analysis has confirmed that HRT has the potential to improve the quality and length of life in any woman but this fact is more applicable following hysterectomy

- We suggest a practical guideline on how health professionals can ensure that women, who would benefit most from HRT, do receive the treatment

Endocrine changes after hysterectomy and oophorectomy

Hysterectomy

Following hysterectomy with ovarian conservation there is an immediate but transient drop in plasma oestrogen levels. This is due to the surgical manipulation of the ovaries resulting an acute reduction in blood flow. Apart from this, plasma oestrogen levels remain unchanged in premenopausal women for at least 12 months following hysterectomy. At that time ovarian histology begins to demonstrate features of relative hypoxaemia and decreasing follicular reserves.[10] The effect of these early structural changes is not clinically evident because of the large functional reserve of the ovaries. If this process continues unabated it results in the manifestation of premature ovarian failure within a few years.

Long-term follow-up (after at least 2 years) shows that plasma FSH levels in young (<44 years) hysterectomized women are higher than in age-matched controls[11] (Figure 2). This is more common in women suffering from hot flushes and represents an impending ovarian failure. The plasma oestrogen levels may initially remain normal with raised FSH but subsequently fall in 25–50% of women. As the most likely cause of premature ovarian failure is decreased blood flow, it is likely to affect the function of ovarian stroma, resulting in a fall of plasma

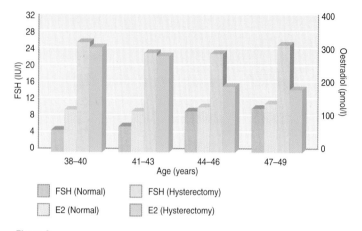

Figure 2
Plasma oestradiol and FSH levels in normal and hysterectomized women of premenopausal age (Adapted from reference 11).

testosterone level as well. These endocrinological changes are seen usually within 2–5 years of surgery but are more liable to develop with longer intervals.[5,6]

Oophorectomy

Premenopausal women who undergo bilateral oophorectomy have more abrupt endocrinological changes. The plasma oestrogen levels fall within 24 hours to values that are 80% below the mean follicular phase levels but similar to those observed after natural menopause.[12] Removal of the ovaries after the menopause results in unaltered plasma oestrogen levels (Figure 3). This is because postmenopausal ovaries make a minimal contribution to the circulating oestrogen, which arises mainly from aromatization of adrenocortical androgens in the peripheral fat.[13,14]

Bilateral oophorectomy in premenopausal women also causes a significant decrease in the plasma testosterone level, owing to the loss of ovarian stroma. Plasma testosterone falls by 30% of the premenopausal range and is significantly lower than that after natural menopause[12] (Figure 3). A relatively lower degree of fall in the testosterone level in comparison to that of oestrogen, is due to the continued extra-ovarian synthesis of testosterone in the adrenal cortex and body fat. In postmenopausal women the ovary is not a defunct endocrine organ, but contributes 50% of the testosterone and 30% of the androstenedione in the circulation.[14,15] Indeed, the ovarian stroma may increase with higher gonadotrophin stimulation, resulting in a higher testosterone level than that before menopause. When the ovaries are removed from postmenopausal women there is a significant fall in circulating levels of testosterone[14] (Figure 3). Thus, testosterone replacement should be considered following oophorectomy, irrespective of whether it is performed before or after the natural menopause.

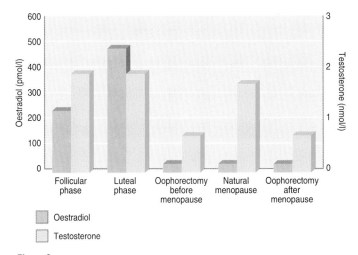

Figure 3
Plasma oestradiol and testosterone levels before and after spontaneous menopause and bilateral oophorectomy.

Indications of HRT after hysterectomy

Pre-existing ovarian failure

As hysterectomy is commonly performed in the 40–49 year age group, the decline in ovarian function often precedes the surgery. These perimenopausal women may have anovulatory cycles resulting in heavy periods, which are often prolonged, irregular and painful. The possibility of impending ovarian failure may not be considered in the presence of periods and even if it is, HRT may be avoided because of the fear of the problem getting worse. Hysterectomy relieves menstrual irregularities, but cannot cure other manifestations of ovarian hormone deficiency. Any further decline in the function of conserved ovaries results in a worsening of cyclical symptoms of bloating, mastalgia, headache, irritability and depression. These symptoms are characteristic of premenstrual syndrome but, in the absence of menstruation, are best termed the *ovarian cycle syndrome*.[16] The diagnosis is usually missed because, in the absence of menstruation, the cyclical pattern of these symptoms may not be recognized. Indeed, they tend to be referred to as vague and inconsistent complaints, probably due to an emotional setback following hysterectomy. *There is a strong case for considering HRT following hysterectomy in all perimenopausal women as they are at higher risk of osteoporosis and cardiovascular disease even in the absence of climacteric symptoms.*

Premature ovarian failure following hysterectomy

The conservation of ovaries at hysterectomy has been advocated as a means of preventing immediate oestrogen loss, but there is accumulating evidence suggesting that retained ovaries may fail prematurely. The incidence of ovarian failure varies between 25–50% of hysterectomized women and can develop at any time, but usually 2–5 years after surgery.[5,6] The age at hysterectomy seems to have no influence on the period of residual ovarian function, but studies have shown that the average age of ovarian failure is four years earlier than in a non-hysterectomized control group.[6] The premature ovarian failure is independent of the indication that leads to hysterectomy, implying that it is the surgery rather than the initial disease that results in to the endocrine changes and the climacteric symptoms. The type of hysterectomy is also irrelevant, but prior tubo-ovarian surgery, resection of ovarian lesions and suturing of the residual ovary are associated with the reduction in the period of future ovarian functioning.

The definite cause of ovarian failure is uncertain, although several possible explanations have been raised.[5,6] These include:

- Interference with ovarian blood supply at the time of surgery
- Disturbance of the normal endometrial-ovarian relationship
- Deficiency of uterine prostaglandin
- Loss of the putative reflex pathway from cervix to pituitary

The compromised ovarian vascular supply resulting from the surgery is the most likely mechanism. Ovaries receive a dual blood supply – through the ovarian artery and the tubal branch of the uterine artery – with a considerable variation in their respective shares (Figure 4). After clamping of the uterine artery, the functioning of residual ovaries depends on the type of blood supply in that individual. This could be the reason for

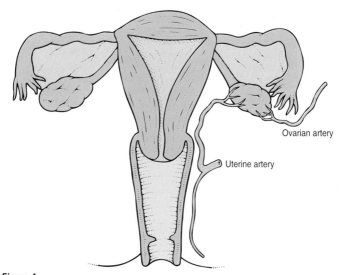

Figure 4
Dual blood supply to the ovary from ovarian and uterine vessels.

ovarian failure in some, but not all, women undergoing hysterectomy. The ovarian veins are devoid of valves and prone to the development of varicosity, which would contribute to the stagnation of ovarian venous flow due to loss of utero-ovarian anastomosis at hysterectomy.[10]

There is rarely any practice of routine follow-up by gynaecologists or general practitioners to enable early diagnosis of this potential iatrogenic ovarian failure after hysterectomy. With the assumption that the conserved ovaries function until the age of natural menopause, the climacteric symptoms are often dismissed or misdiagnosed as psychological illness as a result of hysterectomy. It is unfortunate that these women are often prescribed antidepressants when their problems are so easily treatable with oestrogen. A survey of general practices has shown that among those who are not on HRT following hysterectomy, a quarter of them had FSH levels in the menopausal range in spite of ovarian conservation.[8] Without the vigilance of general practitioners, such women may needlessly be exposed to the risk of cardiovascular disease and osteoporosis.

Bilateral oophorectomy

Approximately 20% of women undergoing hysterectomy for benign conditions have bilateral oophorectomy at the same time. The decision to remove the ovaries is influenced by the indication for hysterectomy and age at the time of surgery. In patients with endometriosis, pelvic congestion syndrome and premenstrual syndrome, oophorectomy is an essential adjunct to hysterectomy for achieving a permanent cure. With other indications for hysterectomy, following full discussion and consent, the ovaries may be removed prophylactically, usually after the age of 40 years. Apart from preventing ovarian cancer, this also avoids any residual ovarian pain and the ovarian cycle syndrome.[16]

As the main argument against bilateral oophorectomy is the consequence of prolonged ovarian hormone deficiency, removal of the ovaries indeed demands HRT immediately after surgery. No matter how beneficial its prophylactic effect, oophorectomy cannot be justified unless arrangements can be made for long-term HRT. Such a clear-cut need for HRT is in many ways preferable to the uncertainty or false assurance with continued function of the residual ovaries. However, in reality, a large number of women who undergo bilateral oophorectomy never take HRT or do so only for a short while after surgery. A survey of general practices in the UK has shown that HRT use in such women is only 30%, even under the age of 40 years.[8] The apparent failure to provide long-term oestrogen therapy in such an obvious high risk population must be seen as a major practical problem surrounding prophylactic oophorectomy before the menopause.

Types, routes and dosage of HRT

Type of hormones

The main differences in the type of hormone replacement therapy given to women who have had hysterectomy with or, without bilateral oophorectomy, compared to non-hysterectomized women, are:

- Progestogen is not required along with oestrogen
- Supplementary testosterone is often needed

In women with a uterus, progestogen is given either cyclically or continuously for protection against endometrial proliferation, but this often results in PMS-like symptoms such as depression, irritability, headache, mastalgia and loss of libido.[7] The fact that hysterectomized women can use oestrogen without progestogen should improve compliance to HRT because of the absence of side-effects. Oestrogen is usually adequate for controlling climacteric symptoms and for protection against the long-term consequences of the natural or surgical menopause. In some women, however, oestrogen alone may not be effective particularly in the relief of lethargy, loss of libido, depression and headache; these symptoms usually respond to the addition of testosterone.[17] The need for testosterone replacement is common following oophorectomy, due to the loss of ovarian androgens.[18]

In premenopausal women the main circulating oestrogen is 17β-oestradiol, which is eventually metabolized to oestrone and oestriol. As the purpose of HRT is to revert the hormonal state to that which existed before menopause, the oestrogens most widely used are the so-called *natural* ones – oestradiol, oestrone and oestriol. Conjugated equine oestrogen is derived from pregnant mares' urine and is mainly composed of oestrone sulphate (50–60%) and many other equine oestrogens. Oestradiol may be replaced using all routes – oral, transdermal, subcutaneous or vaginal – but equine oestrogen is only available for oral and vaginal routes. Synthetic oestrogens, such as ethinyl oestradiol and mestranol, are many times more potent than natural oestrogen and should not be used as HRT following menopause as they may be associated with increased side-effects with prolonged use.

Routes of administration

Subcutaneous implants

Hormone pellet implantation is the most convenient and straightforward route of administration following hysterectomy. It is placed in the wound at the time of hysterectomy followed by subcutaneous insertion every six months. Inserting an implant is a quick, easy and safe office procedure which may be carried out by any practitioner. This is performed under local anaesthesia and the site of choice is the lower part of the anterior abdominal wall, or the upper outer quadrant of the buttock. Initially the trocar and cannula are pushed through a 5 mm skin incision into the subcutaneous fat. The hormone pellet is then inserted down the cannula with the plunger to bury it about 2–3 cm away from the site of entry.

Subcutaneous implantation has the convenience of prolonged duration of action, resulting in excellent compliance as patients do not have to remember to take tablets or apply patches (Table 1). The additional side-effects of other routes, such as gastrointestinal symptoms with tablets and skin irritation with patches, can also be avoided. It has the advantage over oral therapy of avoiding the *first-pass* effect of liver on oestrogen. This results in a physiological ratio of oestradiol/oestrone and also allows a higher bioavailability of oestradiol. It also avoids

	Advantages	Disadvantages
Subcutaneous implant HRT	Compliance Physiological E2 : E1 ratio No first pass hepatic effect Relatively uniform and higher plasma level Testostertone may be given	Minor surgical procedure Pain and swelling at implant site Rejection or expulsion Dose not flexible in short term 'Tachyphylaxis'
Transdermal HRT	Physiological E2 : E1 ratio No first pass hepatic effect No bolus effect Dose flexible No surgery	*Patches:* Adhesion problem Skin reaction: itching and erythema *Gel:* Self overmedication Skin reaction, messy
Oral HRT	Familiar Inexpensive Dose flexible No surgery	Non-physiological E2 : E1 ratio First pass hepatic effect Bolus effect Low dose and potency Poor compliance Gastrointestinal side-effects

Table 1
Advantages and disadvantages with different routes of HRT.

oral oestrogen-induced prothrombotic effects on the clotting system and other potentially adverse metabolic effects such as renin synthesis and an increase in triglyceride levels. Testosterone can be given along with oestrogen via this route.[19]

Plasma hormone levels

One of the great advantages with implants is that the day-to-day levels of plasma oestradiol are remarkably constant (Figure 5). In the long-term, the plasma oestradiol level gradually declines, after peaking between 2 and 4 months after insertion. This results in a recurrence of climacteric symptoms commonly at about 6 months (range 4–12 months), although the hormone levels are usually still within the premenopausal range.[20,21] If another implant is inserted sooner, the hormone level rises even further at the time of each successive implant.[22] Although this phenomenon has resulted in some adverse publicity on the addictive nature of HRT, the problem

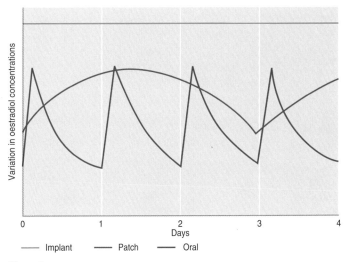

Figure 5
Short term variation in plasma oestradiol levels with different routes of oestrogen replacement.

occurs in only 3% of long-term implant users in whom the higher levels of oestradiol do not appear to have any harmful effects.[23] It may even be beneficial, with satisfactory symptom control and a greater skeletal response since there is a significant relationship between plasma oestradiol level and increases in bone density. Hence, *tachyphylaxis*, suggesting ineffective therapy, is an incorrect terminology to describe the condition, as these women continue to respond well to HRT with adequate symptom control and excellent long-term benefits. If high oestradiol levels occur, the correct management is to continue therapy but at a reduced dosage until plasma levels drop back to the physiological range. Complete withdrawal of oestrogen would be unnecessary harsh with the recurrence of intolerable climacteric symptoms.

Transdermal route

For those patients who chose not to have hormone implants there is an increasingly large selection of other routes. Oestradiol can be given transdermally, either by single membrane **matrix patch** or by the older style **reservoir patch**. The patches are applied to the lower half of the body and are changed every 3 to 4 days. The commonest problem is a skin reaction, which may result in itching and erythema and, rarely, blistering and ulceration. Constant wearing of a patch may also prove to be embarrassing and there may be adhesion problems in hot weather. These side-effects are minimal with matrix patches, which adhere better, are less irritant and are cosmetically more acceptable.

Oestrogen gel is another transdermal option – this has been available in Europe for many years and has recently been released in the UK. The colourless and odourless gel is rubbed into the skin of the inner thigh or upper arm on a daily basis, leaving no residue on the surface. It should improve compliance in patients who find patches unacceptable because of skin irritation and allergy. However, few patients develop skin rash with gel and some consider it "messy".

The transdermal route avoids the first-pass effect of oestrogen on the liver, and so only a tenth of the dose is needed to achieve the same hormone levels and therapeutic effects of a standard oral dose. The other advantages are similar to those of implants – better physiological pharmacokinetic distribution, maintenance of the premenopausal oestradiol/oestrone ratio, and absence of prothrombotic effects of oral HRT. The advantages of the transdermal route over implants are the avoidance of the minor surgical procedure, and the scope for changing the dosage much more rapidly according to the clinical response. One of the limitations of the transdermal route is that testosterone cannot currently be given either by patches or gel, although it is expected that this will be possible in the near future.

Plasma hormone levels

With the transdermal route, plasma oestradiol levels are more stable than oral replacement but may still vary more than 150% during the 3–4 day lifespan of a single patch[24] (Figure 5). There is also an inter-subject variability in hormone absorption of 35–55%.[25] The patches are designed to deliver a steady dose of oestrogen through the skin and doses cannot be increased by changing them more frequently. However, if symptom control is inadequate, the patient may *self-medicate* with more patches or a larger dose of gel which would result in a supraphysiological level of plasma oestradiol.

Oral route

Oral therapy is the most easily accepted and convenient route for many patients, but the lowest available dose may not achieve the required hormone levels. Regardless of the type of oestrogen used, during intestinal absorption it is converted to the less potent form, oestrone, resulting in a reversal of the premenopausal oestradiol/oestrone ratio of 2:1. Further metabolism during the first-pass through the liver inactivates 35–95% of the absorbed oestrogen.[26] Thus an oral dose of oestrogen has to be substantially higher than a dose administered via a non-oral route to achieve similar therapeutic effects. There is also an inter-subject variability in hormone absorption which results in a fluctuation in the oestradiol level of 40–130%.[27] With problems of reduced bioavailability and inter-subject variability in absorption, the standard dose of oral oestrogen is frequently inadequate for complete symptom relief and skeletal protection.

Plasma hormone levels

Oral therapy leads to unstable plasma hormone levels. Within hours of ingestion, a large bolus of oestrogen appears in the systemic circulation resulting in a peak concentration within 4–8 hours. The plasma level then declines rapidly to almost pre-treatment value within 12 hours of intake (Figure 5). In practice, this may not be important in the majority of HRT users but may be responsible for inadequate therapeutic response in some.

With the oral route the liver receives an oestrogen bolus after each dose, the significance of which is debatable. It may be advantageous to avoid the hepatic impact of oral oestrogen in women with labile hypertension, hypertriglyceridaemia or previous thromboembolism due to the potential for altering renin, lipid and clotting factors. On the other hand, with stronger hepatic influence oral oestrogen may have a more powerful effect on lipid metabolism and hence on cardiovascular protection. Severe nausea is one of the rare side-effects produced by only modest doses in which case it is not possible to elevate the plasma level with larger doses.

Dosage of hormones (Table 2)

The conventional practice with HRT is to start at the lowest available dose and increase as required according to alleviation of the patient's symptoms. Following a premature menopause, this may not be appropriate as a relatively higher dose of oestrogen is usually required to attain the physiological oestrogen level in the younger age group. This is more valid

	Symptom relief		Bone protection	
	Minimum	Adequate	Minimum	Adequate
Conjugated oestrogen	0.625 mg	1.25 mg	0.625 mg	1.25 mg
17β oestradiol	1–2 mg	≥2 mg	2 mg	≥2 mg
Oestradiol valerate	1–2 mg	≥2 mg	2 mg	≥2 mg
Oestradiol patch	25 μg	50–100 μg	50 μg	50–100 μg
Oestradiol gel	1 mg	≥3 mg	3 mg	≥3 mg
Oestradiol implant	25 mg	50–75 mg	50 mg	50–75 mg

Table 2
The daily doses of oestrogen for symptom relief and bone protection after hysterectomy in premenopausal women.

after bilateral oophorectomy as the usual hormone production from the ovarian stroma is also lacking. In clinical practice many younger patients who are started on lower doses of oestrogen following bilateral oophorectomy still experience severe menopausal symptoms, and over 75% require a higher dose of HRT.[4,28] More than half of these women need to change the type and dose of HRT at least twice and some up to seven times before achieving satisfactory control. This will reduce the patient's confidence in the treatment and threaten compliance. It would seem to be prudent to use an effective higher dose of oestrogen from the outset following bilateral oophorectomy.

Plasma oestradiol levels

Plasma oestradiol levels fluctuate during the course of an ovarian cycle, with an average of 200–250 pmol/l in the mid-fol-licular phase and 400–500 pmol/l in the mid-luteal phase. In order to bring the level back to this premenopausal range, the choice of dose and route of oestrogen replacement is important. Low-dose oral or transdermal oestrogen is usually unable to achieve the average physiological levels. A higher dose of oral or transdermal oestrogen is required to attain the mid-follicular range[29–31] and an implant of oestradiol (50–75 mg) can reproduce the mid-luteal levels of plasma oestradiol.[32] The plasma FSH levels are also suppressed to the premenopausal range with intermediate and higher oestrogen doses (Figure 6).

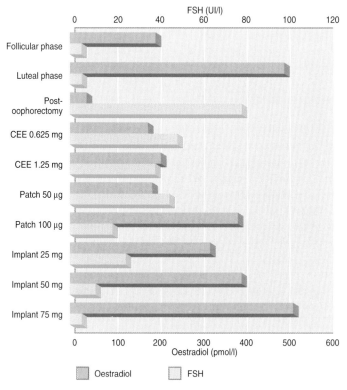

Figure 6
Plasma oestradiol and FSH levels with different doses and routes of replacement in relation to the normal range in an ovarian cycle (adapted from references 29–32).

Plasma oestradiol levels between 200 and 350 pmol/l coincide with the optimal feeling of well-being in most users, depending on their symptoms.[33] The lower oestradiol level obtained from oral or low dose patches is usually effective for the treatment of vasomotor symptoms, insomnia and vaginal dryness. Severe symptoms such as tiredness, headache, depression, loss of libido and bone pain often need the higher dose patches or implants. A relatively higher dose of oestrogen is also required to suppress the cyclical headache, irritability, depression and mastalgia which results from the declining function of the residual ovaries.[19]

Bone loss may be prevented in the majority of women if the plasma oestradiol level is maintained above 200 pmol/l, but to achieve an *increase* in bone density a plasma level of around 350 pmol/l is required. Women with low bone mass may benefit from an oestrogen implant or higher dose patch because of its anabolic effect in improving bone density by enhancing new bone formation.[32]

With regards to the **lipid balance**, there is no dose-effect relationship and little additional clinical benefit is achieved by using a more potent oestrogen regimen.

To obtain both adequate symptom control and protection against osteoporosis, the plasma oestradiol level should ideally be around 250 pmol/l, similar to the mid-follicular phase level. However, the dose of HRT may need to be changed in individuals with oestrogenic side-effects, poor symptom control or sub-optimal bone response.

Relief of climacteric symptoms

Hysterectomized women report both higher frequency and increased severity of climacteric symptoms than do normal women of similar age (Table 3). This is not only limited to those undergoing bilateral oophorectomy but is also seen after ovarian conservation (Figure 7). This results in an increased frequency of consultations with doctors, who should be alert to the presence of oestrogen deficiency symptoms, especially in those who would normally be considered *too young* to have these complaints.

After hysterectomy and bilateral salpingo-ophorectomy the early complaints are vasomotor disturbances. These are perceived by 50% of all patients even before leaving the hospital and by the majority (over 90%) within 6 weeks after surgery. However, these symptoms resolve spontaneously within 6 months in 60% of sufferers and within 5 years in 90%. Thus with time the other oestrogen deficiency symptoms such as depression, loss of libido, and generalized tissue atrophy become the predominant complaints[12] (Figure 8).

With ovarian conservation, the climacteric symptoms develop prematurely, usually after an interval of 2–5 years, and may affect 25–50% of all women undergoing hysterectomy.[5,6,11] During long-term follow-up patients primarily report the atypical symp-

Characteristic symptoms	
Triad	Hot flushes; Night sweats; Vaginal dryness

Non-specific symptoms	
Vasomotor instability	Headache; Migraine; Insomnia; Palpitation; Breathlessness; Faintness
Psychological symptoms	Depression; Anxiety; Panic attack; Irritability; Restlessness; Agoraphobia; Loss of confidence; Forgetfulness; Difficulty in concentrating; Tired on waking; Fatigue; Loss of libido
Urogenital atrophy	Itchy labia; Dyspareunia; Vaginal discharge; Urinary urgency; Dysuria; Urinary incontinence
Generalized connective tissue atrophy	Muscular ache; Bone and joint pain; Pins and needles; Dry thin skin; Brittle nails; Loss of hair

Table 3
Climacteric symptoms.

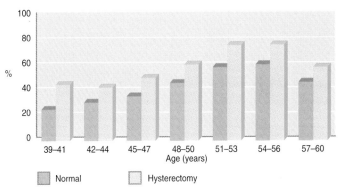

Figure 7
Incidence of climacteric symptoms in normal and hysterectomized women of perimenopausal age (adapted from reference 35).

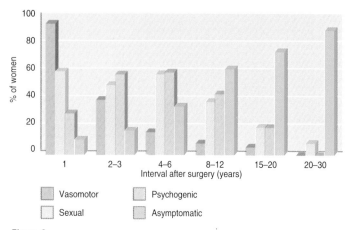

Figure 8
Incidence of climacteric symptoms in oophorectomized women in relation to the time interval after surgery (adapted from reference 12).

toms rather than vasomotor disturbances as the former are usually continuous and often more distressing than the latter.[34,35] However, the atypical symptoms may be difficult to associate with the climacteric unless the presence of vasomotor disturbances is determined. In some patients these symptoms precede hysterectomy and persist in the postoperative period, indicating that sub-optimal ovarian function may remain undetected.[4]

Oestrogen is usually effective in relieving most climacteric symptoms, but a higher therapeutic dose may be necessary for hysterectomized women. The improvement is usually obvious within days and symptoms may be completely eradicated within one cycle. The treatment should be continued for at least 3 months before the dose is increased further, as some women respond gradually. Symptom control is more likely to be effective with the patch and implant, where there is an option of increasing the dosage further if necessary.[30,31] Testosterone replacement should be considered for symptoms that persist in spite of an adequate dosage of oestrogen replacement. The somatic symptom scores are lower with combined oestrogen-testosterone and this is particularly effective in relieving tiredness and headache[17,18] (Figure 9).

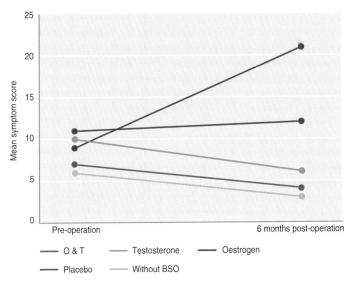

Figure 9
Changes in somatic symptoms with different HRT following hysterectomy and bilateral oophorectomy (Aadapted from reference 18).

Reduced psychological morbidity

In the past, hysterectomy was thought to be responsible for adverse psychological outcome and indeed a *post-hysterectomy syndrome* was recognized.[36] The higher incidence of depression in hysterectomized women was presumed to be due to the surgical treatment, as the preoperative mental state of these patients was unknown. However, several prospective studies have shown that the incidence of depression is higher in women before hysterectomy but postoperatively the mood improves in the majority.[37,38] The incidence and severity of psychiatric disorders in patients before hysterectomy are similar to those of a psychiatric population but postoperatively the rates are closer to those in the general population (Figure 10). It should be no surprise that years of suffering with ineffective medical treatment for heavy periods, chronic pelvic pain, severe premenstrual syndrome and menstrual migraine make women depressed. The improvement in mood following hysterectomy is obviously due to the permanent relief of these debilitating symptoms.

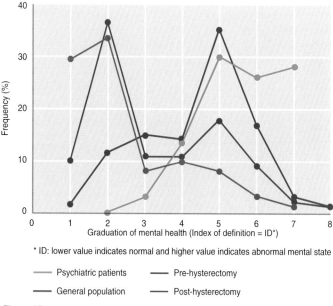

* ID: lower value indicates normal and higher value indicates abnormal mental state

Figure 10
Comparison of the mental health of women undergoing hysterectomy with psychiatric patients and general population (adapted from reference 37).

In some women depression may persist after hysterectomy or develop for the first time postoperatively. This is most likely due to coexisting or subsequent ovarian failure following hysterectomy.[4,39] The aetiological role of declining oestrogen is supported by the occurrence of psychological problems at other times of hormonal flux, such as postnatal depression and premenstrual syndrome. Androgens also have a role in female behaviour, and mood is likely to be affected with removal of their endogenous source following bilateral oophorectomy.[40]

Several double-blind placebo-controlled studies have shown that oestrogen given by any route may improve psychological symptoms following hysterectomy with or without oophorectomy.[41–43] Oestrogen replacement may improve mood by correcting vasomotor instability, insomnia and dyspareunia by a so-called *domino effect* but there is also a dose-dependent mental tonic effect irrespective of any symptoms. Evidently the latter is due to the excitatory effect of oestrogen on the central nervous system, activating the neurones directly by altering the electrical activity and indirectly through neurotransmitters, resulting in the antidepressant effect.

Testosterone replacement in addition to oestrogen may be required to treat any residual depression, particularly following bilateral oophorectomy along with hysterectomy.[17] With combined oestradiol and testosterone implants the incidence of depression drops from 35.6% preoperatively to 3.6% five years after hysterectomy and bilateral oophorectomy.[39] The improvement in psychological symptoms with combined oestrogen and testosterone or testosterone alone is higher than that with oestrogen alone following hysterectomy and bilateral oophorectomy[40] (Figure 11).

Improved sexual outcome

The influence of hysterectomy on sexual function may be variable. There may be improvement in some, no change in many, and deterioration in a small minority of patients.[43,44] An improvement might be expected in individuals whose sexual life has been affected by heavy periods or pelvic pain, which are completely relieved after hysterectomy. There is also an

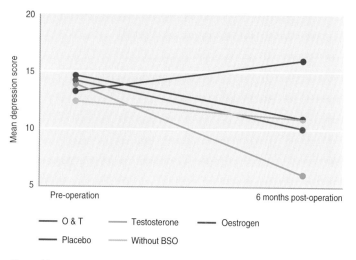

Figure 11

Changes in depression score with different HRT following hysterectomy and bilateral oophorectomy (adapted from reference 30).

enhancement of general well-being following hysterectomy that imparts a positive effect on sexuality. If sexual function is normal before hysterectomy it is most likely to remain unchanged postoperatively. However, an associated ovarian failure can adversely affect sexuality which may either precede hysterectomy or develop later. A positive sexual outcome immediately after hysterectomy followed by deterioration after two years supports a hormonal aetiology rather than a direct effect of surgery.[45] When bilateral oophorectomy is performed, poor sexual function is more common due to the absence of testosterone as well as oestrogen.[43,46]

Ovarian hormone deficiency may affect different aspects of sexuality, such as sexual desire or libido, coital frequency and orgasmic satisfaction. Oestrogen deficiency causes vaginal dryness and impairs peripheral sensory perception, both of which result in dyspareunia. This can reduce sexual frequency and satisfaction, which may lead to secondary loss of libido. Testosterone is involved in the modulation of sex drive and with the decline or loss of the ovarian production there may be a primary loss of libido. Following bilateral oophorectomy, the changes in libido correlate with plasma testosterone rather than oestrogen levels but the coital and orgasmic frequencies are unrelated to the changing levels of circulating hormones.

Oestrogen replacement enhances sexual activity following hysterectomy by relieving vaginal dryness and dyspareunia, without any definite influence on the libido. The positive effect of oestrogen on sexuality is partly due to an improvement in mood and to the relief of menopausal symptoms.[47] Testosterone replacement, either alone or with oestrogen, enhances sexual motivation but has little effect on coitus frequency and orgasmic response[17,48] (Figure 12). Thus, the added effect of testosterone over oestrogen may not always be evident unless loss of libido is a specific complaint.[49]

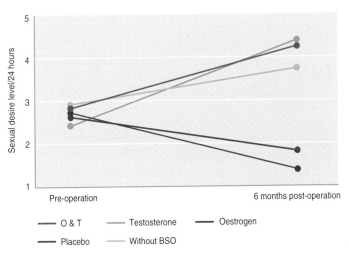

Figure 12
Changes in sexual desire with different HRT following hysterectomy and bilateral oophorectomy (adapted from reference 48).

Improved general health

General health and well-being improve significantly in the majority of patients after hysterectomy.[4,37,38] This results from a marked recovery from fatigue, depression and sexual dysfunction, in addition to the relief of heavy periods and pelvic pain for which the operation has been indicated. The changes are observed within 3 months and are sustained at one year, resulting in an overall improvement in the quality of life. In about 20% of patients, poor general health and well-being persist after hysterectomy; this is due to pre-existing ovarian failure, rather than the indication for surgery.[4] Similarly, ovarian failure following hysterectomy is likely to hamper long-term well-being in spite of initial complete relief of gynaecological symptoms.[34,45]

Oestrogen replacement therapy can prevent a deterioration of general health and-well-being related to ovarian failure. The addition of androgen has a significant effect in improving appetite, well-being and energy levels, especially if the symptoms persist after oestrogen replacement.[17,18] In a prospective study monitoring the differential effect of oestrogen and testosterone following hysterectomy with bilateral oophorectomy, the responses with testosterone alone were similar to the combined oestrogen and testosterone group.[18] They experienced increased well-being, improved appetite and higher energy than the oestrogen-alone and placebo groups (Figure 13). The differential effect is a reflection of the anabolic properties of androgen. *In summary, a routine use of oestrogen and testosterone implants following hysterectomy and bilateral oophorectomy results in better long-term general health and well-being outcome.*[39]

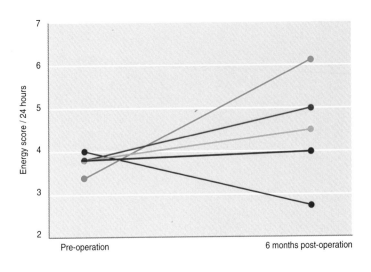

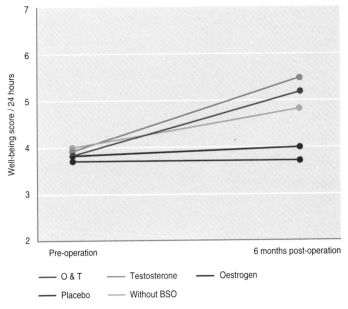

Figure 13
Changes in energy and well-being with different HRT following hysterectomy and bilateral oophorectomy (adapted from reference 18).

Cardiovascular protection

Hysterectomy in premenopausal women is associated with a threefold increased risk of coronary heart disease (CHD) and the deleterious effect has been demonstrated even with ovarian conservation.[50,51] During the ten years following a hysterectomy, it is claimed that there is a 4% probability of developing CHD and 0.4% chance of dying from myocardial infarction.[50] However, others have suggested that CHD occurs predominantly when the ovaries are removed at hysterectomy without giving HRT.[52] The lower the age at surgery, the higher is the risk, so that at the age of 35 years the risk is sevenfold higher than age-matched premenopausal women. Hysterectomized women are also prone to develop **syndrome X**, which manifests with angina pectoris and a positive ECG exercise test without any obvious angiographic coronary obstruction. As the metabolic features are common to those with atheromatous disease it is presumed to be the occult stage of CHD.

It is the early loss of ovarian function that is responsible for the higher incidence of cardiovascular problems. Oestrogen deficiency-induced cardiovascular damage is multifaceted and includes[53,54]:

- Increased arterial resistance
- Adverse changes in circulating lipid and lipoprotein profile
- Alterations in insulin resistance
- Increased body fat in the adverse androgenic distribution
- Changes in haemostatic factors

Hypertension, a known risk factor for CHD, is twice as common in women following hysterectomy with ovarian conservation than in non-hysterectomized controls of similar age.[55]

There is evidence that oestrogen replacement reduces the risk of CHD, but the beneficial effect is proportional to the duration of therapy.[54,56] In women with premature menopause, current use of oestrogen replacement has been reported to nullify the risk of CHD due to ovarian failure, but when oestrogen was discontinued the risk increased by 20%.[57] After the age of 50, the reduction in the risk of CHD among current HRT users was reported to be 50%, and among former users 20%, compared to age-matched individuals who have never taken HRT.[58] The impact of oestrogen was as great, if not greater, in women with high risk factors for cardiovascular disease. The benefit in terms of survival was greatest in women with established CHD, in whom there is an 80% risk reduction in current HRT users.[59]

Oestrogen putatively exerts its beneficial effects on the cardiovascular system in several different ways (Table 4). None of these effects is dose-dependent and little additional benefit is achieved by using a more potent oestrogen regimen. Most of these changes are also independent of the route of oestrogen administration, except for the plasma lipoprotein profile which changes more favourably with the oral route. The preoperative lipid values remain unchanged in premenopausal women if oestrogen replacement is started immediately after hysterectomy and bilateral oophorectomy.[60] The addition of oral test-

Favourable changes in lipid profile	Increases high density lipoprotein (HDL)
	Decreases low density lipoprotein (LDL)
	Decreases lipoprotein (a)
Prevention of atherosclerotic plaque formation	Inhibits cholesterol accumulation
	Prevents LDL-peroxidation
Decrease in arterial resistance	Increases endothelium derived relaxing factor
	Increases endothelial prostacyclin
	Decreases vasoconstrictor endothelin-1
	Decreases Ca-influx in smooth muscle cells
Improvement in cardiac function	Increases cardiac contractility and stroke volume
	Decreases ventricular muscle thickness
Alteration in carbohydrate metabolism	Increases insulin secretion
	Decreases insulin resistance

Table 4
Putative ardiovascular benefits of oestrogen replacement.

osterone has an adverse impact on the circulating lipids and reduces the beneficial effect of oestrogen.[61] This hepatic response is by-passed if a non-oral route is used, and there are no negative effects with testosterone injections or implants.[62]

Prevention of osteoporosis

Women undergoing hysterectomy while still menstruating are more likely to develop osteoporosis than age-matched women who have a spontaneous menopause. This increased risk is due to an earlier onset of accelerated bone loss as a result of the decline in ovarian function following hysterectomy.[63] This problem is often overlooked as the residual ovaries may produce enough oestrogen to avoid vasomotor symptoms but not enough to protect the bones.[64] The rate of bone loss is even faster following bilateral oophorectomy,[65] but if the ovaries are removed after the natural menopause the rate of bone loss is not affected. This confirms that oestrogen deficiency is the single most important causative factor for the increased rate of bone loss.

Bone density has been found to be significantly lower in hysterectomized women with conserved ovaries compared to age-matched non-hysterectomized women, irrespective of their menopausal status.[63,64] In women who have had bilateral oophorectomy the bone density is even lower than those whose ovaries were conserved at hysterectomy (Figure 14). Hormone replacement therapy offers long-term protection against bone loss following hysterectomy – bone density in both current and previous users of HRT is higher than in non-hysterectomized postmenopausal women not taking HRT.[63]

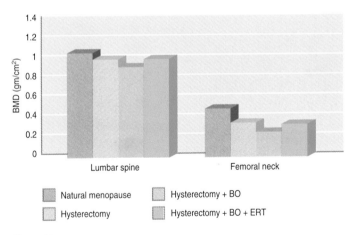

Figure 14
Comparison of bone mineral density between natural and surgical menopause with or without HRT (adapted from reference 63).

A significant proportion of women continue to lose bone despite taking the recommended bone sparing dose of oestrogen (oestradiol valerate 2 mg, conjugated oestrogen 0.625 mg or oestradiol patch 50 µg).[66] It is therefore recommended that either the response is monitored by bone density scans every 2–3 years or a higher initial dose of oestrogen is used (conjugated oestrogen 1.25 mg, oestradiol patch 100 µg or oestradiol implant 50–75 mg).

Oestrogen replacement not only prevents bone loss but can also increase bone mass. The extent of improvement depends on the route and dose used. There is an annual increase in bone density of 2% with oral HRT, 2–3.5% with patches and 6–10% with implants (Figure 15). There is a significant correlation between the plasma oestradiol levels achieved and the percentage increase in bone density, which explains the dose response of oestrogen replacement.[67] Oestradiol implants produce higher oestradiol levels than other preparations and

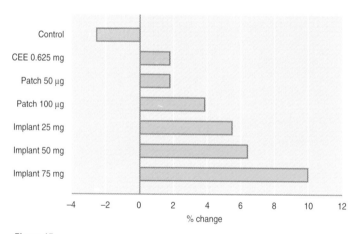

Figure 15
Changes in bone mineral density in a year with different doses and routes of HRT.

therefore lead to a greater therapeutic skeletal response. Women who had a low bone density at baseline have a greater percentage increase with oestrogen replacement. Therefore there is no truth in the view that women over 60 or many years post hysterectomy are *too old* or *too osteoporotic* for HRT.

It has been suggested that androgen has the potential for improving bone mass and bone mineral content, mainly by a direct anabolic effect but also by peripheral conversion to oestrogen. This is supported by the fact that a higher circulating level of androgen is related to a lower incidence of osteoporotic fracture. Following hysterectomy and bilateral oophorectomy, combined oral oestrogen and testosterone replacement has shown a better response in terms of bone density compared to oestrogen alone.[61] Experience with the combined oral preparation containing methyl testosterone is limited as it is not licensed in the UK. With subcutaneous implants the anabolic effect of testosterone on bone is likely to be greater but this has not yet been convincingly demonstrated due to a lack of long-term data.[68]

Risk of breast cancer

The main concern about long-term HRT is the possible increased risk of breast cancer. This is based on the knowledge that the factors leading to prolonged ovarian activity, such as early menarche, late menopause and nulliparity or late first pregnancy, are associated with an increased risk of breast cancer. Conversely, with premature menopause the risk is reduced as the oestrogenic stimulation of breast tissue is minimized. Thus, hysterectomy with or without bilateral oophorectomy in premenopausal women decreases the risk of breast cancer, possibly by curtailing ovarian function at a critical period. The use of HRT in these women up to the age of 50 may increase the risk slightly but it is still lower than in women with normal ovarian function[69,70] (Figure 16). It is therefore inappropriate to extrapolate the risk of long-term HRT after the natural menopause to relatively younger hysterectomized women with premature ovarian failure.

After the age of 50, any increased risk of breast cancer with HRT in hysterectomized women is similar to that after the natural menopause. The large number of studies addressing this issue have been evaluated by several meta-analyses, with a general agreement that short-term (less than 5 years) use of oestrogen does not increase the risk of breast cancer. Two of

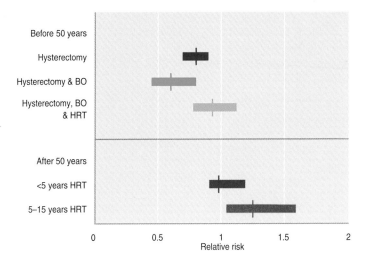

Figure 16
Relative risks of breast cancer following hysterectomy, oophorectomy and HRT (adapted from references 69–71).

the four meta-analyses published to date show that prolonged use (in excess of 8–15 years) gives a duration exposure risk of 25–30% above control[71] (Figure 16). Confusion remains, however. One recent report demonstrated no increased risk irrespective of the duration of use,[72] but another showed increased risk after 5 years.[73] The dose of HRT or route of administration does not appear to affect the risk of breast cancer.

Any excess risk of breast cancer may be due to prolonged stimulation of breast tissue with oestrogen. It could, on the other hand, be a surveillance or detection bias as a result of the increased surveillance that these women receive and the occasional difficulty in making a precise histological diagnosis of cancer or atypical hyperplasia in an oestrogen stimulated organ.[7] This would result in a greater proportion of early stage tumours being detected – this is reflected in the significantly better prognosis and decreased mortality from breast cancer in patients who received oestrogen therapy prior to the diagnosis. The improved longevity following breast cancer treatment among oestrogen users has been confirmed in four out of five papers addressing this issue.[73–75]

Advice for HRT users

Women receiving HRT should be educated regarding breast awareness and advised to seek professional advice should there be any change in their breasts. They should have regular breast examination during clinic visits and mammograms every 3 years from the age of 50. In women taking HRT there is no advantage in having mammograms more frequently than is recommended by the UK national screening programme. In younger women, routine mammograms are unnecessary as they are less sensitive due to the abundance of glandular tissue. If a breast swelling is detected it is useful to perform a mammogram and ultrasound scan to confirm the diagnosis. When breast cancer is diagnosed, HRT should be discontinued because of the uncertainty about any cause-effect relationship, but may be recommended later depending upon the clinical circumstances.

Previous breast cancer

Past history of breast cancer is traditionally regarded as a contraindication to HRT because of the fear of precipitating a relapse. However, it would seem reasonable to use HRT when the quality of life is severely affected by debilitating climacteric symptoms or in the presence of a higher risk of osteoporosis and cardiovascular disease. This recommendation is more appropriate in patients with a lower risk of recurrence and after prolonged disease-free survival, but may also be valid if metastatic disease is widespread and life expectancy is relatively short. Each case must be considered individually and the potential risks and benefits should be discussed with the patient and the oncologist before HRT is started.

There is now a growing view that the risk of recurrence of breast cancer is not increased with HRT use.[76,77] In at least five reports on HRT use in breast cancer patients, there are indications that the risk of recurrence is lower and survival is improved when compared to a matched control group not taking HRT.[71] In some of these studies a continuous high dose of progestogens has been used along with oestrogen, as this has been suggested to be as beneficial as tamoxifen in advanced breast cancer. However, there is insufficient evidence to recommend combined oestrogen and progestogen replacement in hysterectomized breast cancer patients. With the possibility of poor compliance due to progestogenic side-effects, it seems that unopposed oestrogen is the best option at present if there are strong clinical reasons to consider HRT.

Thromboembolism

Contrary to previous opinions, it has recently been reported that the risk of venous thromboembolism (VTE) is increased two- to fourfold in current HRT users.[78,79] The risk appears to be highest at the start of therapy and reduces subsequently in long-term users. In a low-risk population this may result in one extra case of deep vein thrombosis in 5000 users and one extra case of pulmonary embolism in 20 000 users per year. With such a rare occurrence of, and low mortality from VTE, the benefits of HRT still outweigh the risks. This minimal increase in the risk of thromboembolism may be explained by minor changes in the clotting screen with HRT. With oral oestrogen there is a reduction in fibrinogen, increased factor VII and reduction in anti-thrombin III. Avoiding the first-pass hepatic effect by using a non-oral route reduces any potential thrombogenic risks even further as there are no changes in coagulation, fibrinolysis or platelet function.

In patients with active deep vein thrombosis or pulmonary embolism, HRT should be avoided. The relevance of a past history of VTE during hormone use depends on specific circumstances. If the episode was associated with a recognized risk factor such as trauma, surgery, pregnancy or postpartum, then HRT is not contraindicated. In cases of spontaneous onset or recurrent episodes while on the oral contraceptive pill, HRT should be withheld until inherent abnormalities of fibrinolysis or coagulation are excluded. If HRT is prescribed to high-risk individuals, non-oral preparations are preferable. There is no need to stop HRT prior to elective surgery in the absence of proven thrombotic tendency, such as anti-thrombin III or protein C deficiency.

Endometriosis

Hysterectomy is undertaken as the definitive treatment for endometriosis, but the risk of symptom recurrence is six times greater, and the risk of repeat operation eight times higher, unless bilateral oophorectomy is also performed.[80] With the therapeutic need for removal of ovaries these patients require HRT to prevent the consequences of premature menopause. However, there is a theoretical risk of progression or reactivation of endometriosis which has led to a practice of delaying HRT for 6–12 months after surgery to allow atrophy of any residual endometriotic deposits. A recent study has found that there is no advantage in delaying HRT as a means of avoiding recurrence of endometriosis, and so such patients suffer unnecessarily from severe climacteric symptoms following surgery.[80] Continuous combined oestrogen and progestogen replacement has also been suggested to maintain atrophy within the residual foci of endometriosis. However, the fear of recurrence has been shown to be unjustified with no need for intervention following long-term oestradiol and testosterone replacement.[81] This could be due either to the absence of cyclical progestogens, the atrophic effect of testosterone, or the lower sensitivity and concentration of hormonal receptors in the endometriotic deposits. Thus, unopposed oestrogen therapy may be prescribed with apparent surgical removal of all endometriotic areas. In cases where the completeness of the excision is in doubt, it may be advisable to use supplementary testosterone or progestogen along with oestrogen replacement.

Endometrial cancer

Oestrogen replacement is traditionally contraindicated in women who have been treated for endometrial cancer because of the fear of recurrence. This belief has arisen from the known association of unopposed oestrogen with a two- to eightfold increased risk for endometrial adenocarcinoma.[82] In practice, recurrence is rarely a problem as the majority of endometrial cancers are in the early stage, well-differentiated and node negative, and are completely *cured* with hysterectomy. Unopposed oestrogen may therefore be given safely to patients with prognostically favourable endometrial cancer without compromising their long-term survival. This is also the case with endometrial cancer induced by oestrogen replacement, as these are well-differentiated and usually in early stage.[83] Indeed, there are good (although uncontrolled) data to show that disease-free survival after surgery for endometrial cancer is greater if oestrogen therapy is given.[84,85] A recent case–control study has shown that the improved outcome of endometrial cancer in the oestrogen-treated group may be related to case selection. Patients placed on oestrogen replacement postoperatively are usually younger, with early stage and grade of tumour, and have less severe depth of invasion.[86] There is, however, no evidence that oestrogen replacement decreases the disease-free interval or increases the risk of recurrence in stage I and II endometrial cancer. There is a higher incidence of obesity and hypertension in patients with endometrial cancer, and so they are at an increased risk of coronary heart disease and should not be denied the putative cardiovascular benefits of oestrogen replacement. In advanced stages or with residual disease it is appropriate to withhold oestrogen replacement at least for 3–5 years. High doses of progesterone alone may be useful in these patients for the prevention of recurrence and also provide some relief from hot flushes and sweats.

Prescribing practice and compliance

HRT indicated for long-term use

In women with premature ovarian failure following hysterectomy, HRT should be continued at least until the age of natural menopause. Following this essential period, they should be counselled about the use of prophylactic long-term HRT and the decision to continue further will depend upon their own response. As these women are already stable on therapy there should be no need to change the dose or type of replacement after the age of 50. Compliance with long-term HRT following hysterectomy should be excellent in the absence of withdrawal bleeding and progestogenic side-effects (Figure 17), the two most common reasons for poor acceptance and discontinuation of the treatment. Higher rates of acceptability and satisfaction with HRT are to be expected with improved well-being following hysterectomy.

Current practice

A survey of general practices in the UK has shown that only a quarter of hysterectomized women receive HRT. The rate is little different after bilateral oophorectomy, even in women under the age of 40 years. The mean duration of HRT use in women who had a bilateral oophorectomy is only two years.[8]

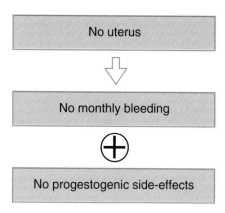

Figure 17
Improved HRT compliance after hysterectomy.

A survey organized by the National Osteoporosis Society reported that HRT awareness is low among hysterectomized women. Of all the respondents who had had a hysterectomy in the previous 5 years, almost two-thirds claimed never to have received any advice about HRT at the time of surgery. Half of these women were not using HRT and 5% of them were not even aware whether their ovaries had been removed at the time of hysterectomy.

There are sporadic reports that indicate a relatively higher HRT uptake rate (70%) than the national average, but even in these studies 15–25% of patients did not receive HRT after bilateral oophorectomy.[87,88] In the gynaecological endocrinology clinic both the uptake and long-term compliance of HRT following hysterectomy and bilateral oophorectomy has been over 90% in women under the age of 40 years.[28] In our own experience with routine use of oestradiol and testosterone implants the continuation rate is 97% after 2–5 years.[39] It is the rate of uptake rather than compliance that is most likely to constrain the use of HRT following hysterectomy.[88] Patient satisfaction has been reported to be higher if follow-up takes place in a dedicated HRT clinic, whether this is in the general practice or at the hospital.[28,88]

Reasons for poor prescribing practice and compliance

Presumed contraindications (Table 5)

There are very few absolute contraindications, but ill-informed medical opinion and unfounded scare stories in the media are the main reasons for not prescribing or taking HRT. In patients with ischaemic heart disease, cerebrovascular accidents, diabetes or hypertension, HRT is often incorrectly avoided. It is well proven that oestrogen is not only safe but in fact can also improve the prognosis of these diseases. The cardiovascular benefits of oestrogen in women who suffer from these conditions are greater than those in healthy women. Thus, these conditions and their risk factors are positive indications for HRT rather than contraindications.

Ischaemic heart disease	Hypertension
Past cerebrovascular accident	Past venous thromboembolism
Superficial thrombophlebitis	Varicose vein
Diabetes	Obesity
Heavy smokers	Migraine
Hepatobilliary problems	Otosclerosis

Table 5
Presumed contraindications of HRT.

There are other conditions, such as migraine, otosclerosis and melanoma, where oestrogen is not contraindicated as there is no definite evidence of any detrimental effect. There is no evidence of any deterioration of liver function tests with HRT but it may be wise to administer oestrogen by a non-oral route in women with liver disease and cholelithiasis (Table 6). Myths about presumed contraindications and side-effects of HRT have arisen because of the failure to discriminate between the potency and action of natural and synthetic oestrogen. This has led to the unfounded extrapolation of oral contraceptive pill data to the HRT information sheets. Incorrect information on the pharmaceutical Data Sheets is a significant factor for the failure to advise HRT by the doctor and the lack of compliance on the part of the patient if HRT has been prescribed.

Acute myocardial infarction	Current venous thromboembolism
Undiagnosed breast lump	Deficient thrombolysis
Active breast cancer	Severe active liver disease
Advanced endometrial cancer	Severe fluid retention

Table 6
True contraindications of HRT.

Incorrect type and dose of HRT

Many clinicians will use the lowest possible dose of oral oestrogen, and as a result some women may still suffer from climacteric symptoms following hysterectomy in spite of taking low-dose HRT. Testosterone supplementation is often not used, which can result in the refractory symptoms of headache, depression, poor libido, tiredness and sub-optimal general well-being. The lack of efficacy resulting from inadequate dose and inappropriate type of HRT may lead to dissatisfaction and discontinuation of the treatment. A higher dose of oestrogen, a more effective route, and the addition of testosterone may be needed for complete symptom control and thereby better compliance with HRT.

Lack of proper follow-up

A further reason for discontinuation of HRT is that there is often inadequate communication between the gynaecologist, the patient and the general practitioner. The patient may be unaware of the importance of HRT following hysterectomy. She may not have been told or remembered whether her ovaries were removed at the time of surgery. The gynaecologist usually discharges the patients after 6 weeks of surgery expecting that the general practitioner will prescribe the HRT. The general practitioner may be under the impression that the patient is receiving HRT from the hospital or may even be uncertain whether an oophorectomy has been performed. As a result of such misunderstanding, the patient may not receive HRT after the initial postoperative dose.

Practical guidelines to improve HRT compliance

The need for long-term HRT following hysterectomy should be emphasized at the stage when the decision of surgery is taken. Before discharging the patient from the hospital the gynaecologist must liaise with the general practitioner regarding follow-up of the patient for HRT. Therapy should be reviewed every 6 months to ensure continued compliance. The dose, type and route of HRT should be altered if there is poor symptom control or side-effects. Those who continue to experience problems even after a change should be referred to a specialist menopause clinic for stabilization. After this stage follow-up may be carried out by the general practitioner, but good communication and continued access to the specialist menopause clinic should be maintained if any problems develop in future.

Health professionals should be particularly vigilant about the possibility of premature failure of the residual ovaries when dealing with hysterectomized patients. The diagnosis of ovarian failure is straightforward in the presence of typical climacteric symptoms. With atypical complaints it is helpful to enquire about any associated vasomotor symptoms and arrange for a blood test to check FSH and oestradiol levels. An FSH level of more than 20 IU/l with or without an oestradiol level of less than 50 pmol/l is confirmatory of ovarian failure, but is not an essential prerequisite to starting HRT. Many women experience their most severe symptoms because of fluctuations in hormone levels and should not be denied HRT on the basis of pre-menopausal hormone levels.

Ideally, all women who have had hysterectomy with ovarian conservation should be screened annually for ovarian failure. It is easy to identify hysterectomized women in a community as they are the ones who are excluded from the cervical cancer screening list. Two blood tests at a two-week interval are needed to avoid an incorrect diagnosis due to low oestradiol in early follicular phase or high FSH in the mid-cycle. An abnormal hormonal profile confirming ovarian failure is an indication for HRT, even in the absence of any climacteric symptoms. It is also important to identify those women who are not taking HRT following bilateral oophorectomy. Thus all hysterectomized women in a community should be sent a reminder to attend the clinic every 12 months for either a hormone screen or for continuation of HRT.

Conclusion

Quality of life

A well-performed hysterectomy in a woman with long-standing symptoms of heavy painful periods can transform her life. Similarly, other cyclical symptoms such as premenstrual syndrome, menstrual migraine and perimenopausal depression will all be cured by hysterectomy and bilateral oophorectomy followed by efficient HRT. While earlier retrospective studies indicated the presence of a *post-hysterectomy syndrome* of tiredness, depression and sexual problems, prospective studies on the effect of hysterectomy have, on the other hand, shown an improvement in these symptoms resulting in a better quality of life. Earlier studies merely demonstrated that women who need hysterectomy are more depressed than the general population, owing to long-standing gynaecological symptoms. However, the possibility of coexisting or subsequent ovarian failure as the cause of poor physical and psychological recovery was not addressed. In reality, the occurrence of depression following hysterectomy and adequate HRT is very rare and limited to those with pre-existing endogenous depression.

Ovaries – to remove or to conserve?

The decision to remove ovaries during hysterectomy is an important one and should be taken after careful counselling and consent from the patient. Such women need long-term hormone replacement by tablets, patches, gels or implants. Frequently they also need testosterone to replenish the missing ovarian androgen, without which the symptoms of depression, loss of energy, loss of libido and poor well-being persist. Such treatment is best administered by hormone implants of 50 mg oestradiol and 100 mg testosterone every 6 months. The continuation rate for this effective treatment has been reported as 97% after 2–5 years, reflecting the fact that these doses produce adequate plasma oestradiol and testosterone levels, resulting in an improved well-being appreciated by the patients. After hysterectomy there is of course no bleeding and no need for progestogen with its frequent side-effects of bloating, breast discomfort, headache and depression. There are other reasons for good compliance.

In patients whose ovaries are conserved there should not be a complacent view that they will continue to function until the normal menopausal age. There is evidence that residual ovaries may fail earlier, although it remains uncertain whether this is due to surgery or whether the symptoms of menorrhagia requiring hysterectomy occur in patients who are already experiencing premature ovarian failure. It is important to recognize that if such patients develop non-specific climacteric type symptoms, which are often cyclical, this may be due to relative oestrogen deficiency from failing ovaries. It is easy to assume that such symptoms are non-hormonal in origin because the ovaries have been left behind and the patient is younger than the expected age. In women with a uterus the climacteric symptoms are at their worst 2–3 years before menopause. This may not be recognized in hysterectomized women who do not have the signal of period irregularities and naturally occurring amenorrhoea. Even in the absence of symptoms the hormone profile should be checked annually, with high FSH being an earlier diagnostic finding than a low plasma oestradiol. Such patients need hormone therapy; any route may be suitable but these patients respond best of all to oestradiol and testosterone implants.

Risks and benefits

Hysterectomized women are at a higher risk of cardiovascular disease and osteoporosis due to prolonged oestrogen deficiency following early ovarian failure. Hormone replacement should therefore be continued long term, which is likely to be more acceptable in the absence of uterus-related side-effects. The main worry associated with long-term HRT is the possible increased risk of breast cancer, but even if this risk is real it is not valid until the age of natural menopause and perhaps 8–10 years after that. Moreover, it is reassuring to note that there are fewer deaths from breast cancer among HRT users than in non-users. The benefits of long-term HRT thus far outweigh the risks. The risks and benefits may be balanced by using HRT for 10 years after the age of 50 to get adequate bone protection and relief from vasomotor symptoms with minimal increased risk of breast cancer. Thus prophylactic HRT becomes cost-effective by improving the quality-adjusted life expectancy in hysterectomized women.

In spite of the well-established immediate and long-term benefits of HRT following hysterectomy, the majority of such patients do not receive this treatment. This is largely due to a lack of follow-up and inadequate communication between the gynaecologist and the general practitioner. The traditional low-dose oestrogen replacement may not be adequate for complete relief of climacteric symptoms and may be discontinued if the patient loses confidence in the treatment. Thus, the potential need for a relatively higher dose of oestrogen and sometimes additional testosterone should be understood following surgical menopause. Fears about the safety of HRT in conditions such as cardiovascular disease, diabetes, hypertension, liver disease, melanoma and otosclerosis have been shown to be unfounded. It is the responsibility of health professionals to clarify the fact that patients with these presumed contraindications would actually benefit from HRT. With correct advice, proper selection of HRT preparation and arrangement for follow-up, there need not be any problem with long-term compliance.

References

1. Coulter A, McPherson K, Vessey M. Do British women have too many or too few hysterectomies? *Soc Sci Med* 1988; **27**:987–994.
2. Studd JWW. Shifting the indications for hysterectomy. *Lancet* 1995; **345**:388–389.
3. Studd JWW. Hysterectomy and menorrhagia. *Baillière's Clin Obstet Gynecol* 1989; **3**:415–424.
4. Carlson KJ, Miller BA, Fowler FJ. The Maine women's health study: I. Outcomes of hysterectomy. *Obstet Gynecol* 1994; **83**:556–565.
5. Riedel HH, Lehman-Willenbrock E, Semm K. Ovarian failure phenomenon after hysterectomy. *J Reprod Med* 1986; **31**:597–600.
6. Siddle N, Sarrel P, Whitehead M. The effect of hysterectomy on the age at ovarian failure: identification of a subgroup of women with premature loss of ovarian function and literature review. *Fertil Steril* 1987; **47**:94–100.
7. Studd JWW. The complications of hormone replacement therapy in post-menopausal women. *J R Soc Med* 1992; **85**:376–378.
8. Spector TD. Use of oestrogen replacement therapy in high risk groups in the United Kingdom. *BMJ* 1989; **299**:1434–1435.
9. Norman SG, Studd JWW. A survey of views on hormone replacement therapy. *Br J Obstet Gynecol* 1994; **101**:879–887.

10. Souza AZ, Fonseca AM, Izzo VM, Clauzet RM, Salvatore CA. Ovarian histology and function after total abdominal hysterectomy. *Obstet Gynecol* 1986; **68**:847–849.

11. Kaiser R, Kusche M, Wurz H. Hormone levels in women after hysterectomy. *Arch Gynecol Obstet* 1989; **244**:169–173.

12. Chakravarti S, Collins WP, Newton JR, Oram DH, Studd JWW. Endocrine changes and symptomatology following oophorectomy in pre-menopausal women. *Br J Obstet Gynecol* 1977; **84**:769–775.

13. Vermeulen A. The hormonal activity of the post-menopausal ovary. *J Clin Endocrinol Met* 1976; **42**:247–253.

14. Judd HL, Judd GE, Lucas WE, Yen SSC. Endocrine function of postmenopausal ovary: concentration of androgens and oestrogens in ovarian and peripheral vein blood. *J Clin Endocrinol Met* 1974; **39**:1020–1023.

15. Adashi EY. The climacteric ovary as a functional gonadotrophin driven androgen producing gland. *Fertil Steril* 1994; **62**:20–27.

16. Studd JWW. Prophylactic oophorectomy. *Br J Obstet Gynecol* 1989; **96**:506–509.

17. Brincat M, Magos AL, Studd JWW et al. Subcutaneous hormone implants for the control of climacteric symptoms. A prospective study. *Lancet* 1984; **i**:16–18.

18. Sherwin BB, Gelfand MM. Differential symptom response to parenteral oestrogen and /or testosterone administration in the surgical menopause. *Am J Obstet Gynecol* 1985; **151**:153–160.

19. Studd JWW, Smith RNJ. Oestradiol and testosteone implants. *Baillière's Clin Endocrinol Metab* 1993; **7**:203–223.

20. Thom MH, Collins WP, Studd JWW. Hormonal profile in postmenopausal women after therapy with subcutaneous implants. *Br J Obstet Gynecol* 1981; **88**:426–433.

21. Barlow DH, Abdalla HI, Roberts et al. Long-term hormone implant therapy: hormonal and clinical effects. *Obstet Gynecol* 1985; **67**:321–325.

22. Ganger K, Cust M, Whitehead M. Symptoms of oestrogen deficiency associated with supraphysiological plasma oestradiol concentration in women with oestradiol implants. *BMJ* 1989; **299**:601–602.

23. Garnett TJ, Studd JWW, Hendrson A et al. Hormone implants and tachyphylaxis. *Br J Obstet Gynecol* 1990; **97**:917–921.

24. Power MS, Schenkel L, Darley PE et al. Pharmacokinetics and pharmacodynamics of transdermal dosage forms of 17β oestradiol: comparison with conventional oral oestrogen used for hormone replacement. *Am J Obstet Gynecol* 1985; **152**:1099–1106.

25. Scott RT, Ross B, Anderson C, Archer DF. Pharmacokinetics of percutaneous oestradiol: a crossover study using gel and transdermal system in comparison with oral micronized oestradiol. *Obstet Gynecol* 1991; **77**:758–764.

26. Dusterberg B, Schmidt-Gollwitzer M, Humpel M. Pharmacokinetics and biotransformation of estradiol valerate in ovariectomized women. *Hormone Res* 1985; **21**:145–154.

27. Kuhnz W, Gansau C, Mahier M. Pharmacokinetics of oestradiol, free and total oestrone in young women following oral administration. *Drug Metab* 1993; **43**:966–973.

28. Reid BA, Ganger KF. Oophorectomy in young women: can it ever be justified? *Contemp Rev Obstet Gynaecol* 1994; **6**:41–45.

29. Utian WH, Katz M, Davey DA, Carr PJ. Effect of premenopausal castration and incremental dosage of conjugated equine oestrogen on plasma FSH, LH and oestradiol. *Am J Obstet Gynecol* 1978; **132**:297–302.

30. Kamel EM, Maurer SA, Hochler MG, Hoffman DI, Rebar RW. Gonadotropin dynamics in women with receiving immediate or delayed transdermal oestradiol after oophorectomy. *Obstet Gynecol* 1991; **78**:98–102.

31. Anderson CHM, Raju SK, Forsling ML, Wheeler MJ. Oestrogen replacement after oophorectomy: comparison of patches and implants. *BMJ* 1992; **305**:90–91.

32. Studd JWW, Holland EFN, Leather AT, Smith RNJ. The dose-response of percutaneous oestradiol implants on the skeletons of postmenopausal women. *Br J Obstet Gynecol* 1994; **101**:787–791.

33. Dupont A, Dupont P, Cusan L et al. Comparative endocrinological and clinical effects of percutaneous oestradiol and oral conjugated oestrogen as replacement therapy in menopausal women. *Maturitas* 1991; **13**:297–311.

34. Schofield MJ, Bennett A, Redman S, Walters WAW, Sanson-Fisher RW. Self-reported long-term outcomes of hysterectomy. *Br J Obstet Gynecol* 1991; **98**:1129–1136.

35. Oldenhave A, Jaszmann L, Everaerd W, Haspels A. Hysterectomised women with ovarian conservation report more climacteric complaints than do normal climacteric women of similar age. *Am J Obstet Gynaecol* 1993; **168**:765–771.

36. Richards DH. A post-hysterectomy syndrome. *Lancet* 1974; **ii**:983–985.

37. Gath D, Cooper P, Day A. Hysterectomy and psychiatric disorder: I. Levels of psychiatric morbidity before and after hysterectomy. *Br J Psych* 1982; **140**:335–342.

38. Ryan MM, Dennerstein L, Pepperell R. Psychological aspects of hysterectomy: a prospective study. *Br J Psych* 1989; **154**:516–522.

39. Khastgir G, Studd JWW. A survey of patient's attitude, experience and satisfaction with hysterectomy, oophorectomy and hormone replacement by oestradiol and testosterone implants. *Obstet Gynecol* 1998 (Submitted).

40. Sherwin BB and Gelfand MM. Sex steroids and affect in the surgical menopause: a double blind cross over study. *Psychoneuroendocrinology* 1985; **10**:325–335.

41. Dikoff EC, Crary WG, Christo M, Lobo RA. Oestrogen improves psychological function in postmenopausal women. *Obstet Gynecol* 1991; **78**:991–995.

42. Best N, Rees M, Barlow D. Effect of oestradiol implant on nonadrenergic function and mood in menopausal patients. *Psychoneuroendocrinology* 1992; **17**:87–93.

43. Nathorst-Boos J, von Schoultz B. Psychological reaction and sexual life after hysterectomy with and without oophorectomy. *Gynecol Obstet Invest* 1992; **34**:97–101.
44. Helstrom L, Lundberg PO, Sorbom D, Backstrom T. Sexuality after hysterectomy: a factor analysis of women's sexual lives before and after hysterectomy. *Obstet Gynecol* 1993; **81**:357–362.
45. Bernhard LA. Consequence of hysterectomy in the lives of women. *Health Care Women Int* 1992; **13**:281–291.
46. Studd JWW, Collin WP, Chakravarti S, Newton JR, Oram D, Parsons A. Oestradiol and testosterone implants in the treatment of psychosexual problems in the post-menopausal women. *Br J Obstet Gynecol* 1977; **84**:314–315.
47. Dennerstein L, Burrows GD, Wood C, Hymann G. Hormones and sexuality: effect of oestrogen and progestogen. *Obstet Gynecol* 1980; **56**:316–322.
48. Sherwin BB, Gelfand MM, Brender W. Androgen enhances sexual motivation in females: a prospective, crossover study of sex steroid administration in the surgical menopause. *Psychosom Med* 1985; **47**:339–350.
49. Burger H, Hailes J, Nelson J, Menelaus M. Effect of combined implants of oestradiol and testosterone on libido in postmenopausal women. *BMJ* 1984; **294**:936–937.
50. Centerwall BS. Premenopausal hysterectomy and cardiovascular disease. *Am J Obstet Gynecol* 1981; **139**:58–61.
51. Palmer JR, Rosenberg L, Shapiro S. Reproductive factors and risk of myocardial infarction. *Am J Epidemiol* 1992; **131**:408–416.
52. Rosenburg L, Hennenkens CH, Rosner B, Belanger C, Rothman KJ, Speizer FE. Early menopause and the risk of myocardial infarction. *Am J Obstet Gynecol* 1981; **139**:47–51.
53. Gruchow HW, Anderson AJ, Barboriak JJ, Sobocinski KA. Postmenopausal use of oestrogen and occlusion of coronary heart disease. *Am Heart J* 1988; **115**:954–963.

54. Stampfer MJ, Colditz GA, Willett WC. Menopause and heart disease: a review. *Ann N Y Acad Sci* 1990; **592**:193–203.

55. Luoto R, Kaprio J, Reunanen A, Rutanen E-M. Cardiovascular morbidity in relation to ovarian function after hysterectomy. *Obstet Gynecol* 1995; **85**:515–522.

56. Stampfer MJ, Colditz GA. Oestrogen replacement therapy and coronary heart disease: a quantitative assessment of the epidemiological,evidence. *Prev Med* 1991; **20**:47–63.

57. Grady D, Rubin SM, Petitti DB et al. Hormone therapy to prevent disease and prolong life in postmenopausal women. *Ann Intern Med* 1992; **117**:1016–1037.

58. Rosenburg L, Slone D, Shapiro S, Kaufman D, Stolley PD, Miettinen OS. Noncontraceptive oestrogen and myocardial infarction. *JAMA* 1980; **244**:339–342.

59. Sullivan JM, Zwagg RV, Lemp GF et al. Oestrogen replacement and coronary heart disease. *Arch Intern Med* 1990; **150**:2557–2562.

60. Erenus M, Kutlay K, Kutlay L. Comparison of the impact of oral versus transdermal oestrogen on serum lipoproteins. *Fertil Steril* 1994; **61**:300–302.

61. Watts NB, Notelovitz M, Timmons MC, Addison WA, Wiita B, Downey LJ. Comparison of oral oestrogen and oestrogen plus androgen on bone density and lipid-lipoprotein profiles in surgical menopause. *Obstet Gynecol* 1995; **85**:529–537.

62. Sherwin BB, Gelfand MM, Schucher R, Gabor J. Postmenopausal oestrogen and androgen replacement and lipoprotein lipid concentration. *Am J Obstet Gynecol* 1987; **156**:414–419.

63. Hreshchyshyn MM, Hopkins A, Zylstra S, Anbar M. Effects of natural menopause, hysterectomy and oophorectomy on lumber spine and femoral neck bone densities. *Obstet Gynecol* 1988; **72**:631–638.

64. Watson N, Studd J, Garnett T, Leather A, Savvas M, Milligan P. Bone loss following hysterectomy with ovarian conservation. *Obstet Gynecol* 1995; **86**:72–77.

65. Pansini F, Bagni B, Bonaccorsi G et al. Oophorectomy and spinal bone density: evidence of higher rate of bone loss in surgical compared with spontaneous menopause. *Menopause* 1995; **2**:109–115.

66. Bouillon B, Burckhardt P, Christiansen C et al. Consensus development conference: prophylaxis and treatment of osteoporosis. *Am J Med* 1991; **90**:107–110.

67. Studd JWW, Savvas M, Watson NR et al. The relationship between plasma oestradiol and the increase in bone density in postmenopausal women after treatment with subcutaneous hormone implants. *Am J Obstet Gynecol* 1990; **163**:1474–1479.

68. Garnett TJ, Studd JWW, Savvas M, Watson NR, Leather AT. The effects of plasma oestradiol levels on the increase in vertebral and femoral bone density following oestradiol and testosterone implants. *Obstet Gynecol* 1992; **79**:768–772.

69. Irwin KL, Lee NC, Peterson HB, Rubin GL, Wingo PA, Mandel MG. Hysterectomy, tubal sterilization and risk of breast cancer. *Am J Epidemiol* 1988; **127**:1192–1201.

70. Meijer WJ, van Lindert ACM. Prophylactic oophorectomy. *Eur J Obstet Gynecol Reprod Biol* 1992; **47**:59–65.

71. Sands R, Boshoff C, Jones A, Studd JWW. Hormone replacement therapy after a diagnosis of breast cancer. *Menopause* 1995; **2**:73–79.

72. Stanford JL, Weiss NS, Voigt LF et al. Combined oestrogen and progestin hormone replacement in relation to risk of breast cancer in middle-aged women. *JAMA* 1995; **274**:137–142.

73. Colditz GA, Hankinson SE, Hunter DJ et al. The use of oestrogen and progestin and the risk of breast cancer in postmenopausal women. *N Engl J Med* 1995; **332**:1589–1593.

74. Hunt K, Vessey M, McPherson K. Mortality in a cohort of long-term users of hormone replacement therapy: an update analysis. *Br J Obstet Gynecol* 1990; **97**:1080–1086.

75. Bergvisk L, Adami HO, Persson I et al. Prognosis after breast cancer diagnosis in women exposed to oestrogen and oestrogen-progestogen replacement therapy. *Am J Epidemiol* 1992; **130**:221–228.

76. DiSaia PJ. Hormone replacement therapy in patients with breast cancer. *Cancer Suppl* 1993; **71**:1490–500.

77. Powels TJ, Hickish T, Casey S et al. Hormone replacement after breast cancer. *Lancet* 1993; **342**:60–61.

78. Daly E, Vessey MP, Hawkins MM et al. Risk of venous thromboembolism in users of hormone replacement therapy. *Lancet* 1996; **348**:977–980.

79. Grodstein F, Stampfer MJ, Goldhaber SZ et al. Prospective study of exogenous hormones and risk of pulmonary embolism in women. *Lancet* 1996; **348**:983–987.

80. Namnoum AB, Hickman TN, Googman SB, Gehlbach DL, Rock JA. Incidence of symptom recurrence after hysterectomy for endometriosis. *Fertil Steril* 1995; **64**:898–902.

81. Henderson AF, Studd JWW, Watson NR. *A Retrospective Study of Oestrogen Replacement Therapy following Hysterectomy for Endometriosis. Proceeding of the ICI Conference on Endometriosis; Sept 1989; Cambridge.* Carnforth: Parthenon Press, 1990:133–142.

82. Rubin GL, Peterson HB, Lee MC, Maes EF, Wingo PA, Backer S. Oestrogen replacement therapy and the risk of endometrial cancer: remaining controversies. *Am J Obstet Gynecol* 1990; **162**:148–152.

83. McGonigle KF, Karlan BY, Barbuto DA, Leuchter RS, Lagasse LD, Judd HL. Development of endometrial cancer in women on oestrogen and progestogen hormone replacement therapy. *Gynecol Oncol* 1994; **55**:126–132.

84. Creasman WT, Henderson D, Hinshaw W, Clarke-Pearson DL. Oestrogen replacement therapy in the patient treated for endometrial cancer. *Obstet Gynecol* 1986; **67**:326–330.

85. Lee RB, Burke TW, Park RC. Oestrogen replacement therapy following treatment for stage I endometrial carcinoma. *Gynecol Oncol* 1990; **46**:189–191.

86. Chapman JA, DiSaia PJ, Osnan K, Roth PD, Gillotte DL, Berman ML. Oestrogen replacement therapy in surgical stage I and II endometrial cancer survivors. *Am J Obstet Gynecol* 1996; **175**:1195–1200.
87. Seeley T. Oestrogen replacement therapy after hysterectomy. *BMJ* 1992; **305**:811–812.
88. Griffiths F, Convery B. Women's use of hormone replacement therapy for relief of menopausal symptoms, for prevention of osteoporosis and after hysterectomy. *Br J Gen Pract* 1995; **45**:355–358.

Index